*Place a special photo here.*

# Baby's First Years

A Keepsake Book

PaRragon.

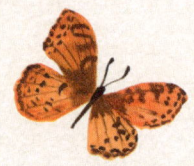

## Dedication

........................................................................
........................................................................
........................................................................
........................................................................

Copyright © 2023 Cottage Door Press, LLC
5005 Newport Drive, Rolling Meadows, Illinois 60008

Illustrated by Rachel Grant

All rights reserved. No part of this publication may be reproduced, stored in a retrieval system, or transmitted, in any form or by any means, electric, mechanical, photocopying, recording, or otherwise, without the prior permission of the copyright holder.

ISBN 978-1-64638-862-2

www.cottagedoorpress.com

Cottage Door Press® and the Cottage Door Press® logo are registered trademarks of Cottage Door Press, LLC.

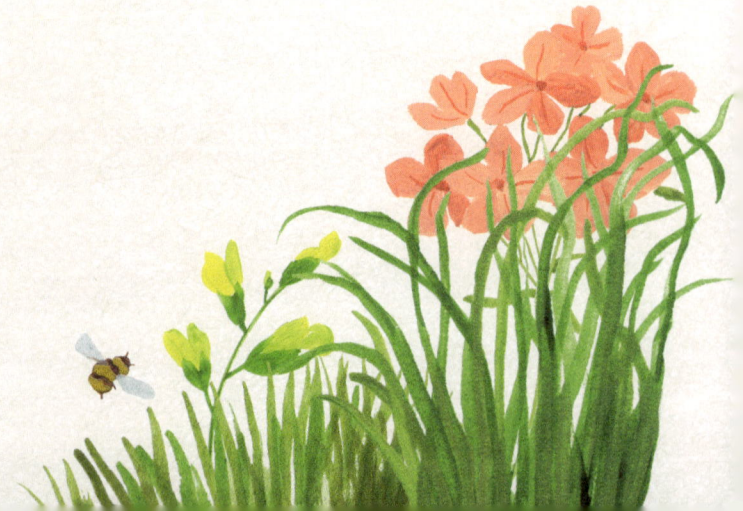

# Contents

| | |
|---|---|
| A Letter to You Before You Are Born | 4 |
| Our Family Tree | 6 |
| About Our Family | 7 |
| The Day You Were Born | 8 |
| Welcome Home | 10 |
| Ten Tiny Fingers and Ten Tiny Toes | 11 |
| Your Name | 12 |
| First Things First | 14 |
| Milestones | 16 |
| One Month | 18 |
| Two Months | 20 |
| Three Months | 22 |
| Four Months | 24 |
| Five Months | 26 |
| Six Months | 28 |
| Seven Months | 30 |
| Eight Months | 32 |
| Nine Months | 34 |
| Ten Months | 36 |
| Eleven Months | 38 |
| Twelve Months | 40 |
| Happy First Birthday! | 42 |
| A Year of You | 44 |
| Wishes for You | 45 |
| You're Two Cool! | 46 |
| Two Terrific Years | 48 |
| Young, Wild, and Three! | 50 |
| Three Years Strong | 52 |
| Favorite Places | 54 |
| Beginning with Books | 56 |
| Animal Friends | 58 |
| Holiday Moments | 60 |
| A Letter to Future You | 62 |

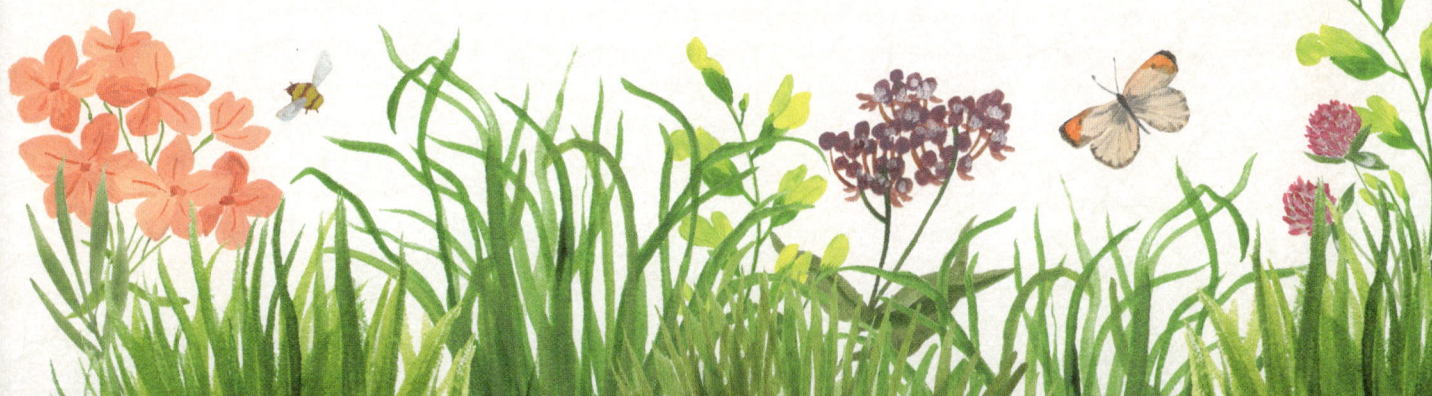

# A Letter to You Before You Are Born

These are our hopes, dreams, wishes, and predictions about future you.

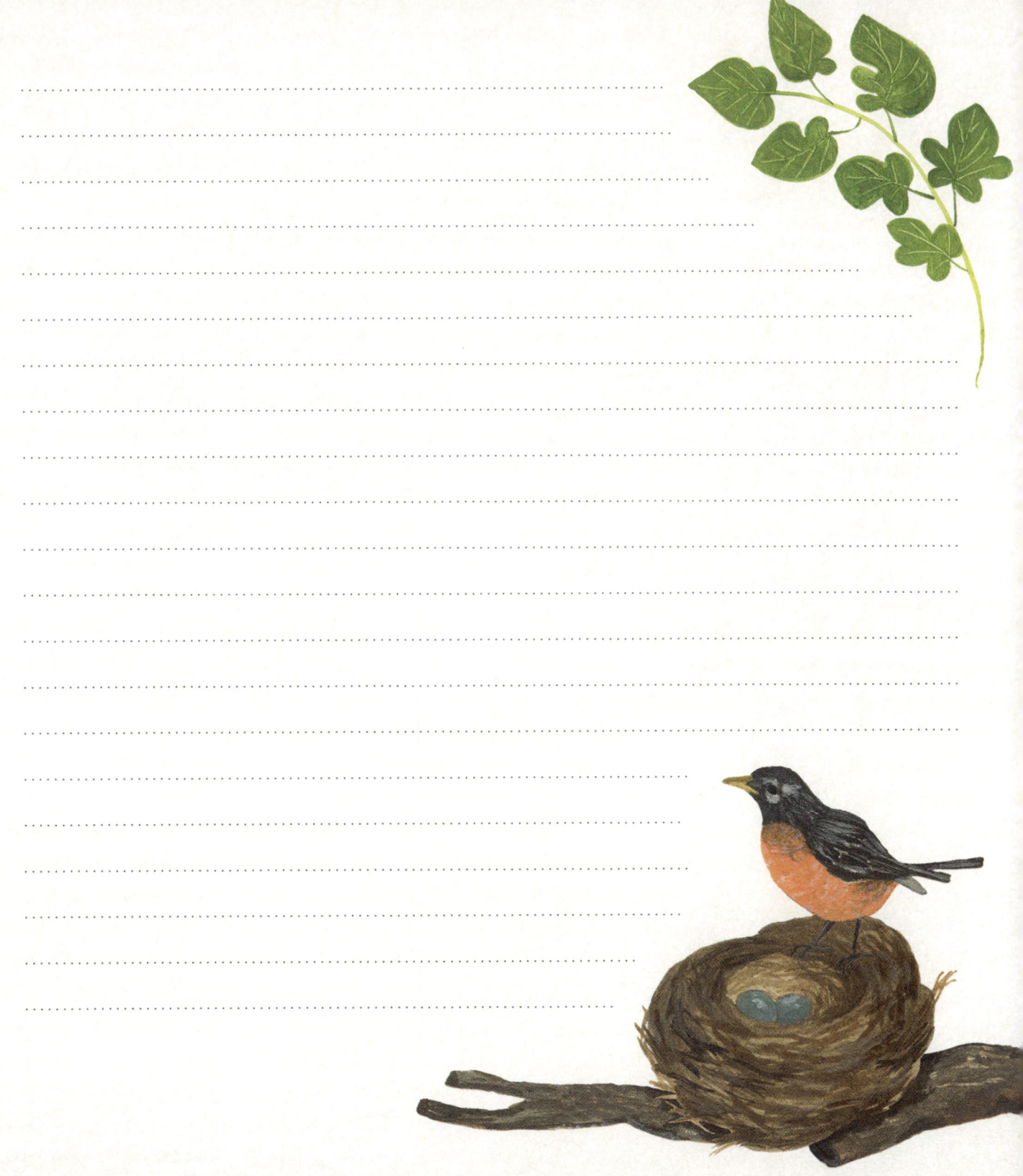

# Our Family Tree

Use stickers to add names to the tree.

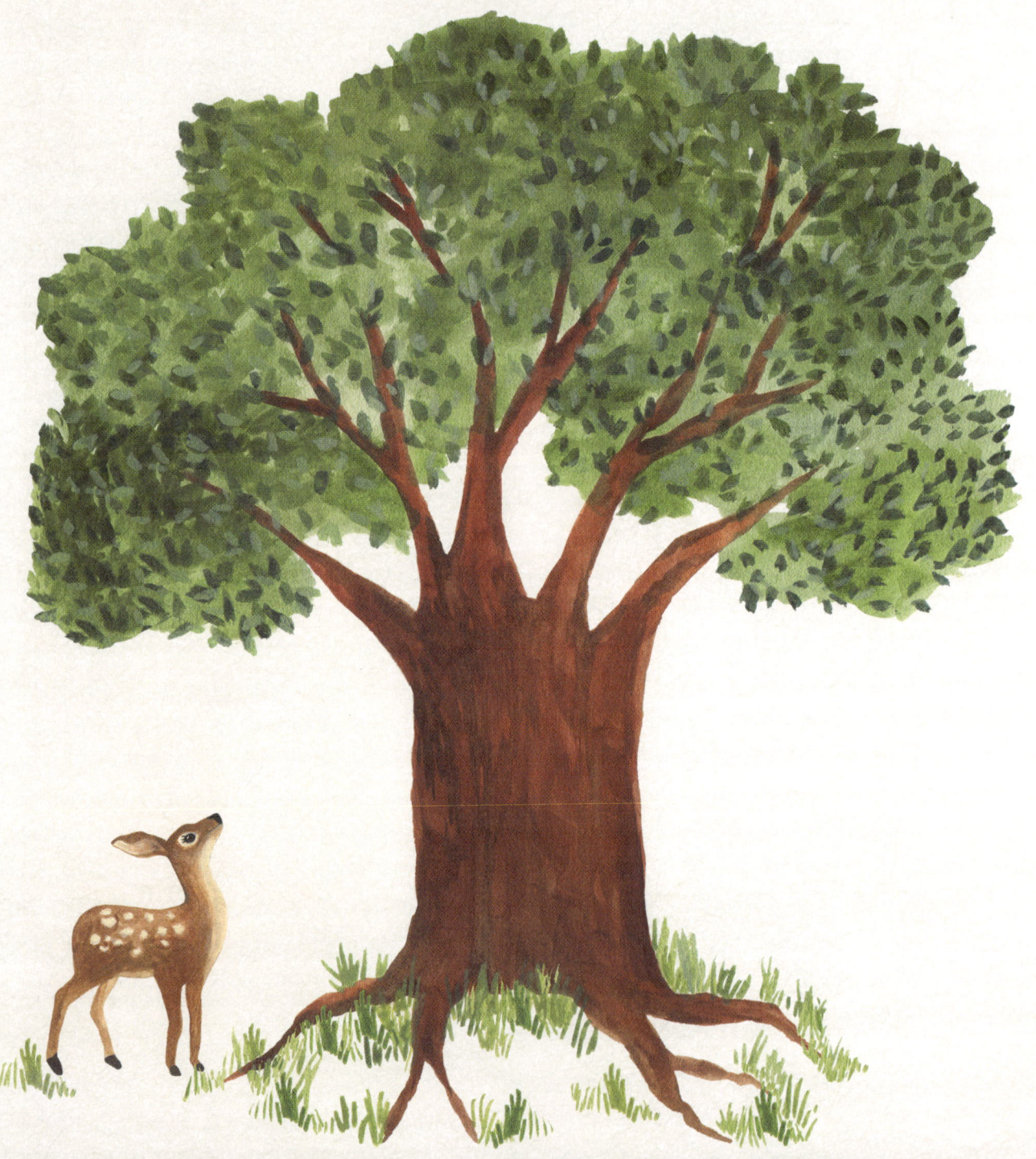

## About Our Family

*A family photo*

More special people we want you to know about:

# The Day You Were Born

## Your Birth Story

*Baby's first photo*

# Ten Tiny Fingers and Ten Tiny Toes

Place baby's handprint and footprint on this page.

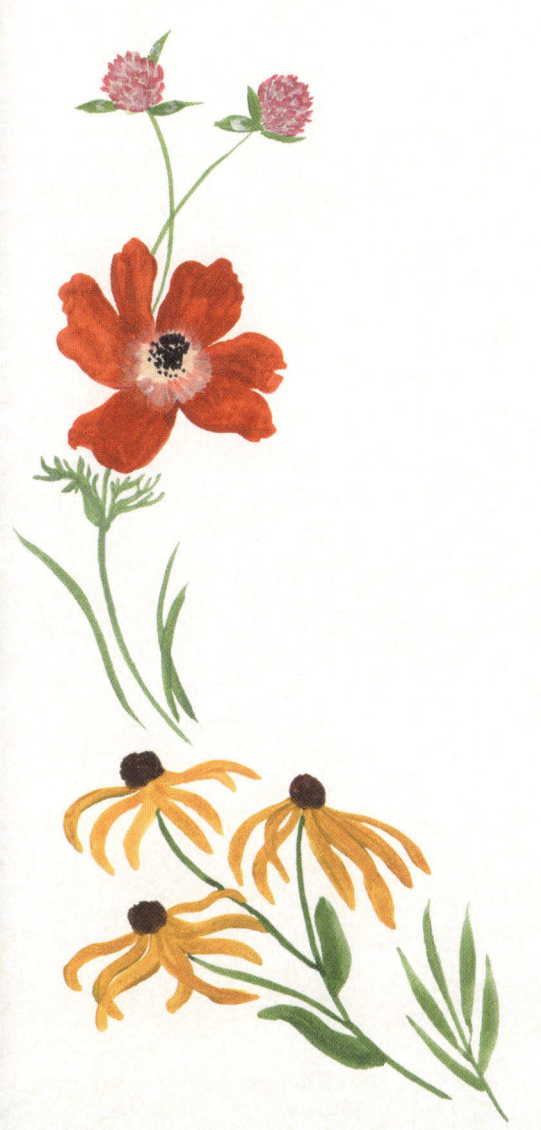
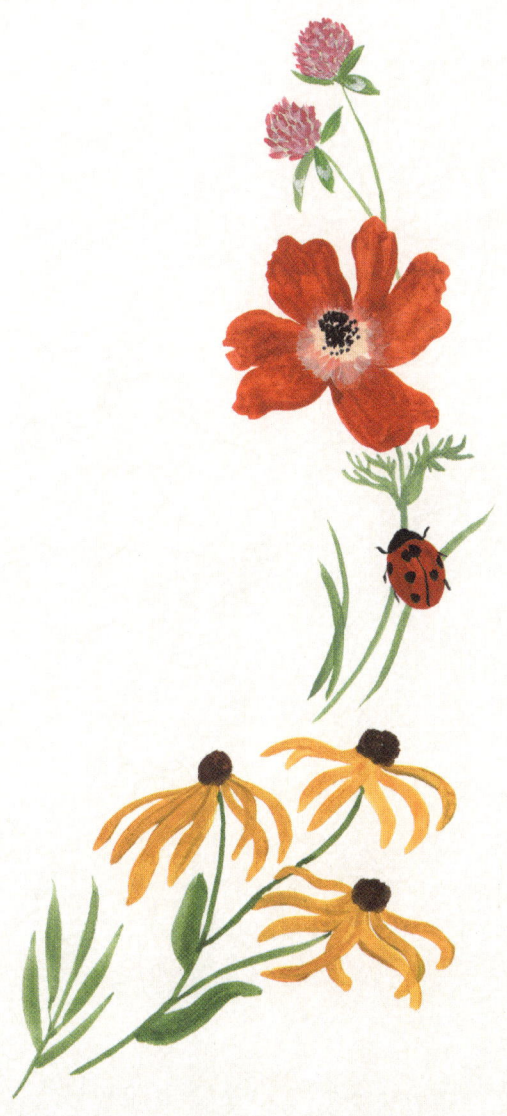

# 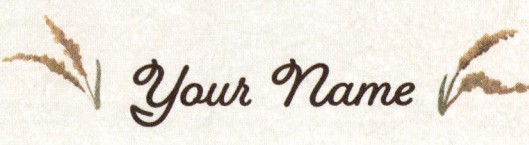 Your Name

Your full name is ..............................................................................................

Your name means ............................................................................................
..................................................................................................................
..................................................................................................................
..................................................................................................................

The inspiration for your name was .....................................................................
..................................................................................................................
..................................................................................................................
..................................................................................................................

You share your name with ................................................................................
..................................................................................................................
..................................................................................................................

Other names we considered were ......................................................................
..................................................................................................................
..................................................................................................................
..................................................................................................................

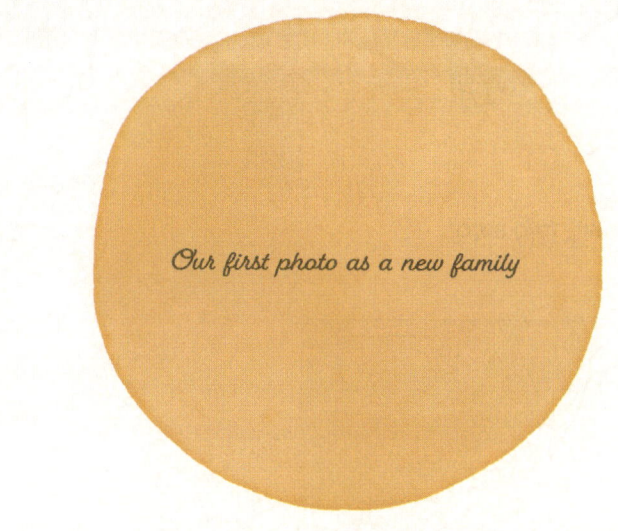

*Our first photo as a new family*

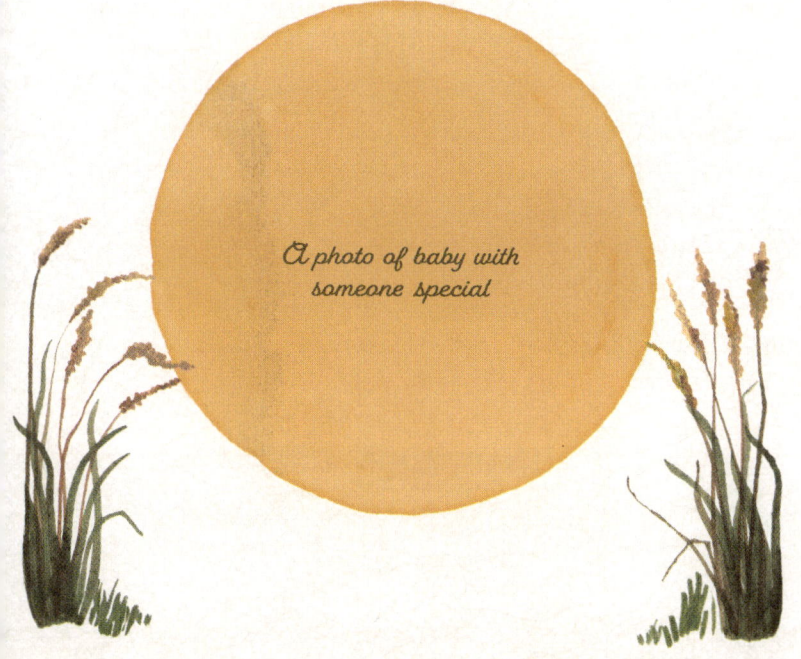

*A photo of baby with someone special*

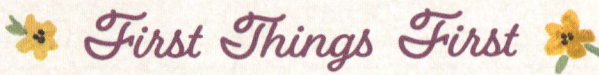

# First Things First

These are some of your most memorable "firsts."

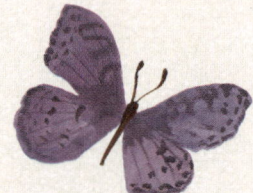

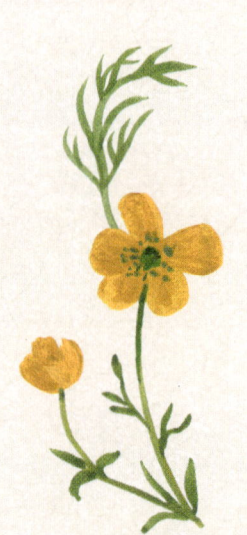

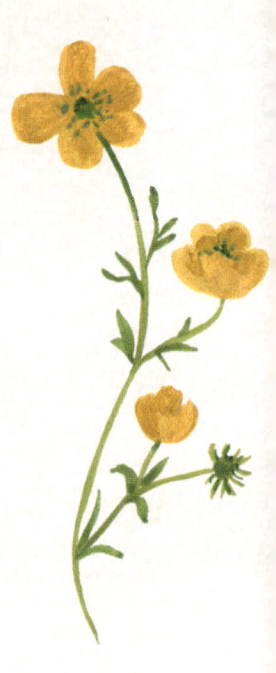

*A photo of a special "first"
(baby's first bath, meeting someone
for the first time, or a first smile)*

..................................................................................................................................
..................................................................................................................................
..................................................................................................................................
..................................................................................................................................
..................................................................................................................................

Your First Solid Food

..................................................
..................................................
..................................................
..................................................

A photo of baby eating
something yummy

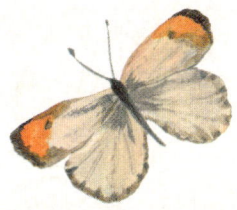

Your First Steps

..................................................
..................................................
..................................................
..................................................

A photo of baby walking

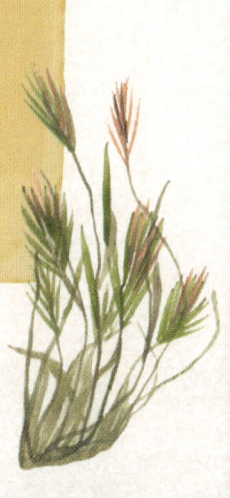

# Milestones

You first smiled ..........................................

Your first bath ............................................

Your first outing ..........................................

You first met your grandparents ..............

Your first doctor's appointment ...............

You first laughed ........................................

You first rolled over ...................................

You first slept through the night .............

You first sat up ...........................................

You first crawled .........................................

You first waved ...........................................

Your first bottle ..........................................

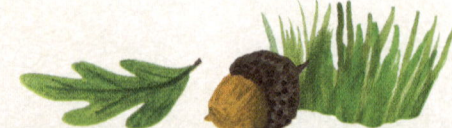

You first stood .................................  You first walked .................................

Your first tooth .................................  Your first word .................................

Your first solid food .........................  Your first haircut ...............................

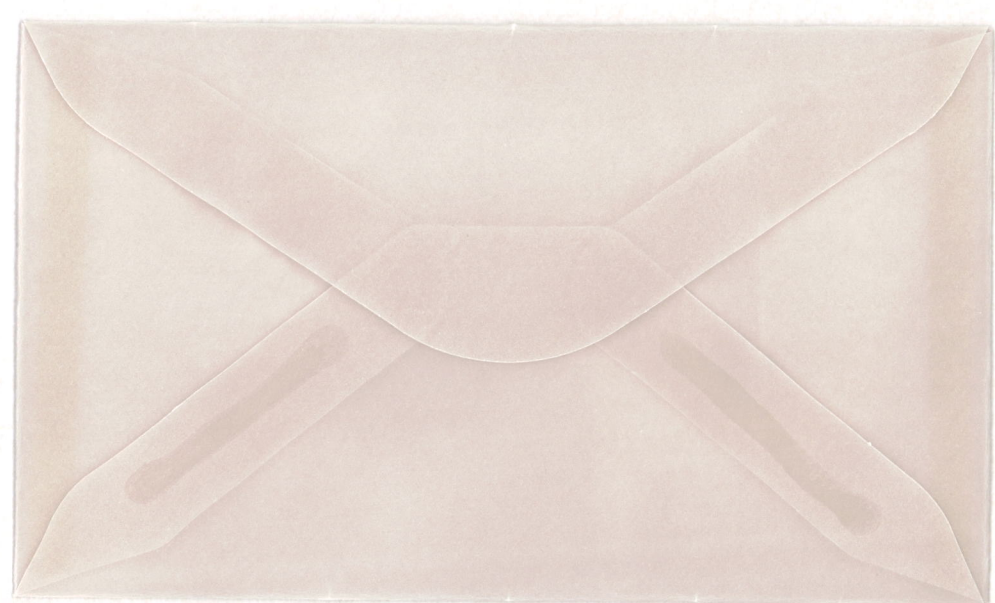

*A lock from baby's first haircut*

# One Month

On .................................................
 you turned one month old!

You weigh .....................................
and are ....................... inches tall.

You love ......................................
..................................................
..................................................
..................................................

*One month old!*

You don't like ............................
..................................................
..................................................
..................................................
..................................................

You can ......................................
..................................................
..................................................
..................................................

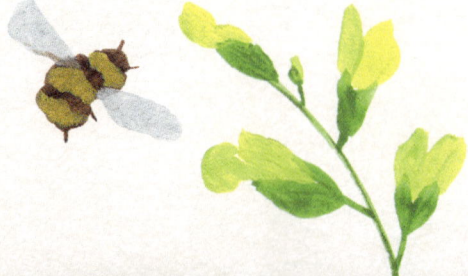

Favorite book: .................................

..............................................................

Favorite food: .................................

..............................................................

Favorite activity: ............................

..............................................................

Favorite song: ................................

..............................................................

Our family's favorite moments with you this month: ..........................

..............................................................

..............................................................

..............................................................

..............................................................

..............................................................

*A favorite one-month memory*

..............................................................

..............................................................

# Two Months

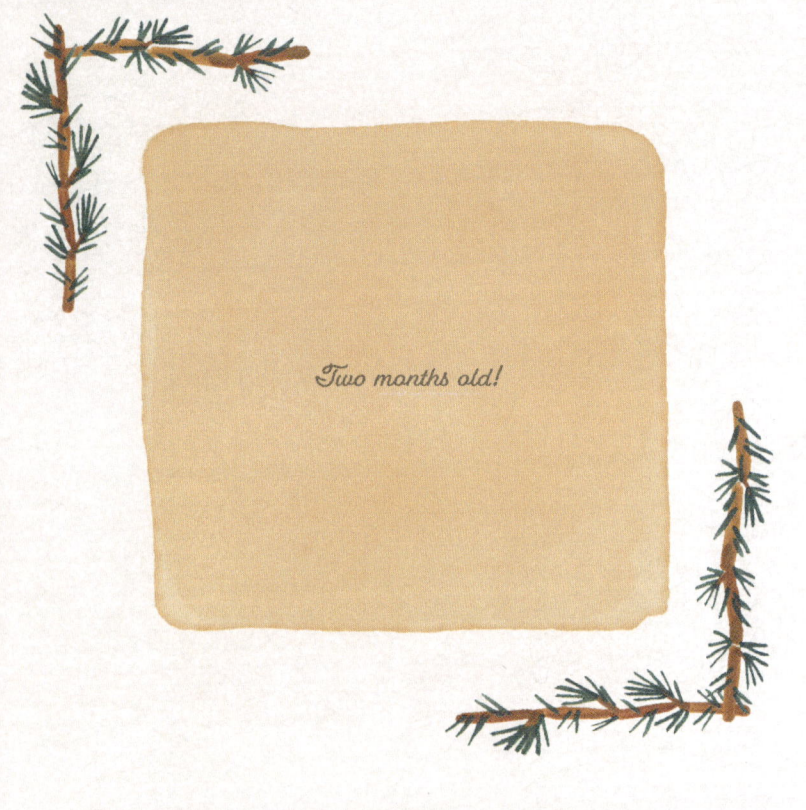

*Two months old!*

On .................... you turned two months old!

You weigh ....................
and are .................... inches tall.

You love ....................
....................
....................
....................

You can ....................
....................
....................
....................

You don't like ....................
....................
....................

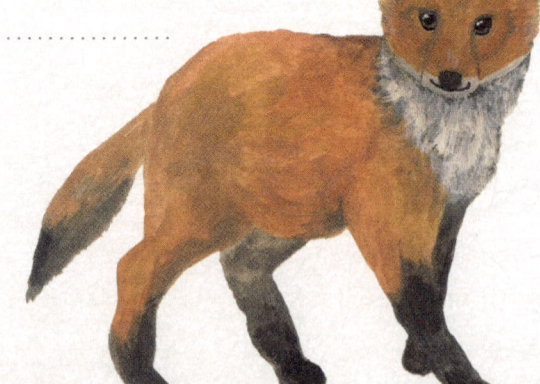

Favorite book: .................... Favorite activity: ....................
........................... ...........................

Favorite food: .................... Favorite song: ....................
........................... ...........................

*A favorite two-month memory*

Our family's favorite moments with you this month:

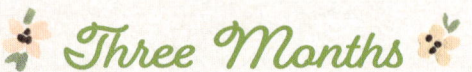
# Three Months

On ............................................................
you turned three months old!

You weigh ...............................................
and are ........................ inches tall.

*Three months old!*

You love ...................................................
................................................................
................................................................

You don't like ..........................................
................................................................
................................................................
................................................................

You can ....................................................
................................................................
................................................................
................................................................

................................................................................................................

................................................................................................................

*A favorite three-month memory*

Favorite book: ............................  Favorite activity: ............................
................................................  ................................................

Favorite food: ............................  Favorite song: ............................
................................................

Our family's favorite moments with you this month: ............................
................................................................................................................

................................................................................................................

# Four Months

On .................................................

you turned four months old!

You weigh ............................

and are ...................... inches tall.

You love ...............................

..............................................

..............................................

..............................................

You don't like ......................

..............................................

..............................................

..............................................

You can ................................

..............................................

..............................................

..............................................

..............................................

..............................................

*Four months old!*

Favorite book: ..................................

Favorite food: ..................................

Favorite activity: ..................................

Favorite song: ..................................

Our family's favorite moments with you this month: ..................................

*A favorite four-month memory*

## Five Months

On .................................................
you turned five months old!

You weigh .................................................
and are ....................... inches tall.

You love .................................................
.................................................
.................................................
.................................................

*Five months old!*

You don't like .......................................
.................................................
.................................................

You can .................................................
.................................................
.................................................
.................................................

Favorite book: ....................................

..................................................................

Favorite food: .....................................

..................................................................

Favorite activity: ................................

..................................................................

Favorite song: ....................................

..................................................................

Our family's favorite moments with
you this month: ..................................

..................................................................

..................................................................

..................................................................

..................................................................

..................................................................

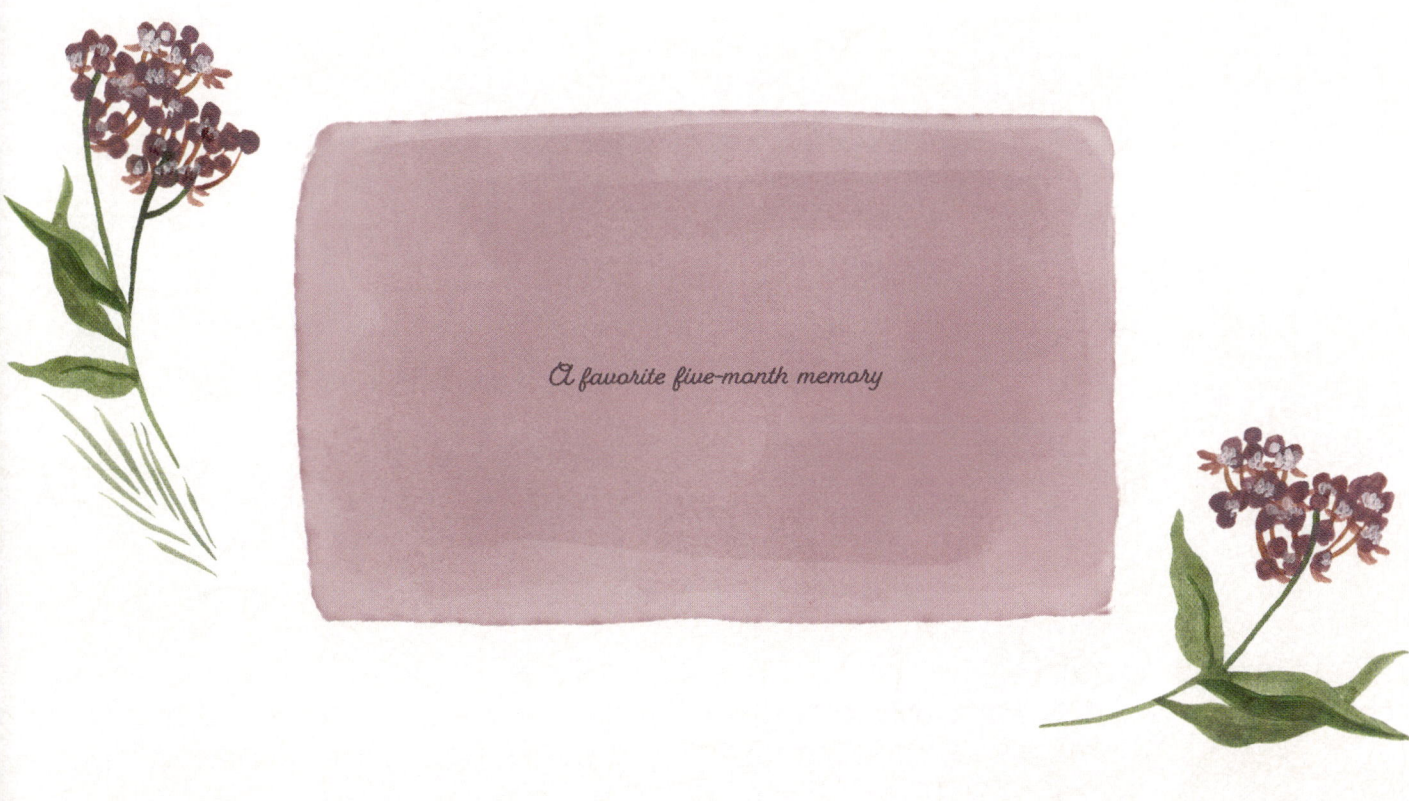

*A favorite five-month memory*

..................................................................

..................................................................

# Six Months

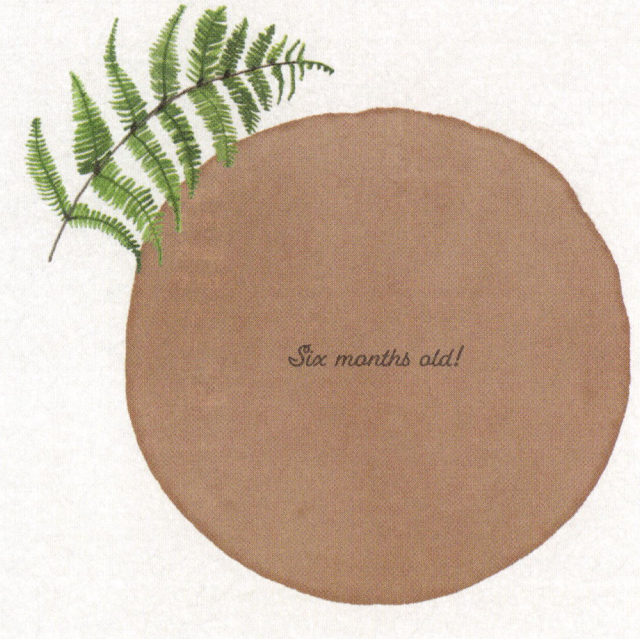

*Six months old!*

On ..........................................
you turned six months old!

You weigh ..................................
and are .................... inches tall.

You love ...................................
..............................................
..............................................
..............................................

You can ....................................
..............................................
..............................................
..............................................
..............................................

You don't like .............................
..............................................
..............................................
..............................................
..............................................

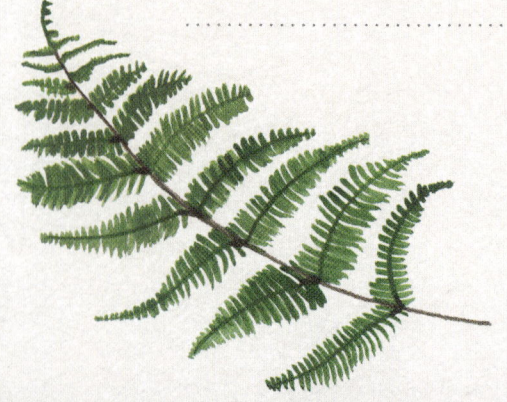
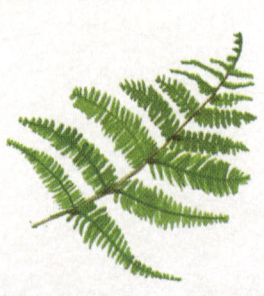

Favorite book: ............................  Favorite activity: ............................
........................................  ........................................

Favorite food: ............................  Favorite song: ............................
........................................  ........................................

*A favorite six-month memory*

........................................................................
........................................................................

Our family's favorite moments with you this month: ............................
........................................................................
........................................................................

# Seven Months

On ............................................... you turned seven months old!

You weigh ...............................
and are ....................... inches tall.

*Seven months old!*

You love ...............................................
................................................................
................................................................
................................................................

You don't like .......................................
................................................................
................................................................
................................................................
................................................................
................................................................

You can ................................................
................................................................
................................................................
................................................................
................................................................
................................................................

*A favorite seven-month memory*

Favorite book: .................................

Favorite activity: ...............................

Favorite food: .................................

Favorite song: ...............................

Our family's favorite moments with you this month: ...............................

# Eight Months

On ............................................... you turned eight months old!

You weigh ...............................
and are ................... inches tall.

You love ...............................................
..........................................................
..........................................................

You don't like ........................
..........................................................
..........................................................
..........................................................

You can ...............................................
..........................................................
..........................................................
..........................................................
..........................................................
..........................................................

*Eight months old!*

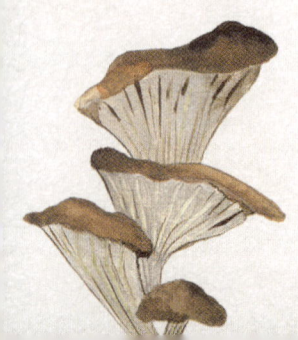
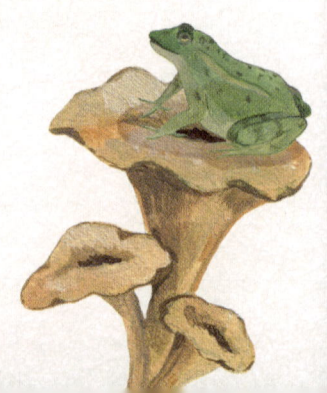

Favorite book: ....................................

............................................................

Favorite food: ....................................

............................................................

Favorite activity: ...............................

............................................................

Favorite song: ....................................

............................................................

Our family's favorite moments with
you this month: ................................

............................................................

............................................................

............................................................

............................................................

*A favorite eight-month memory*

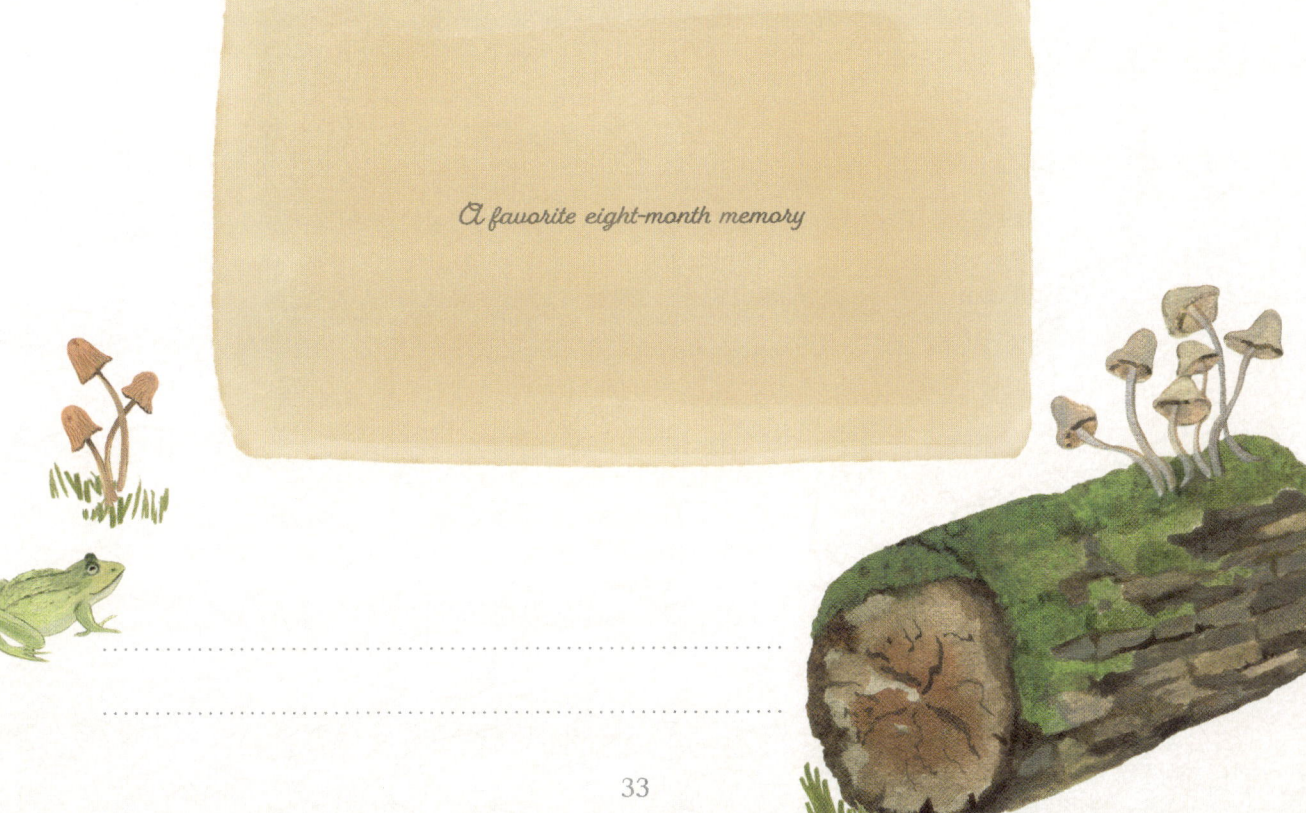

# Nine Months

On ..................................................
you turned nine months old!

You weigh ...................................
and are ......................... inches tall.

You love ..................................................
..................................................
..................................................
..................................................

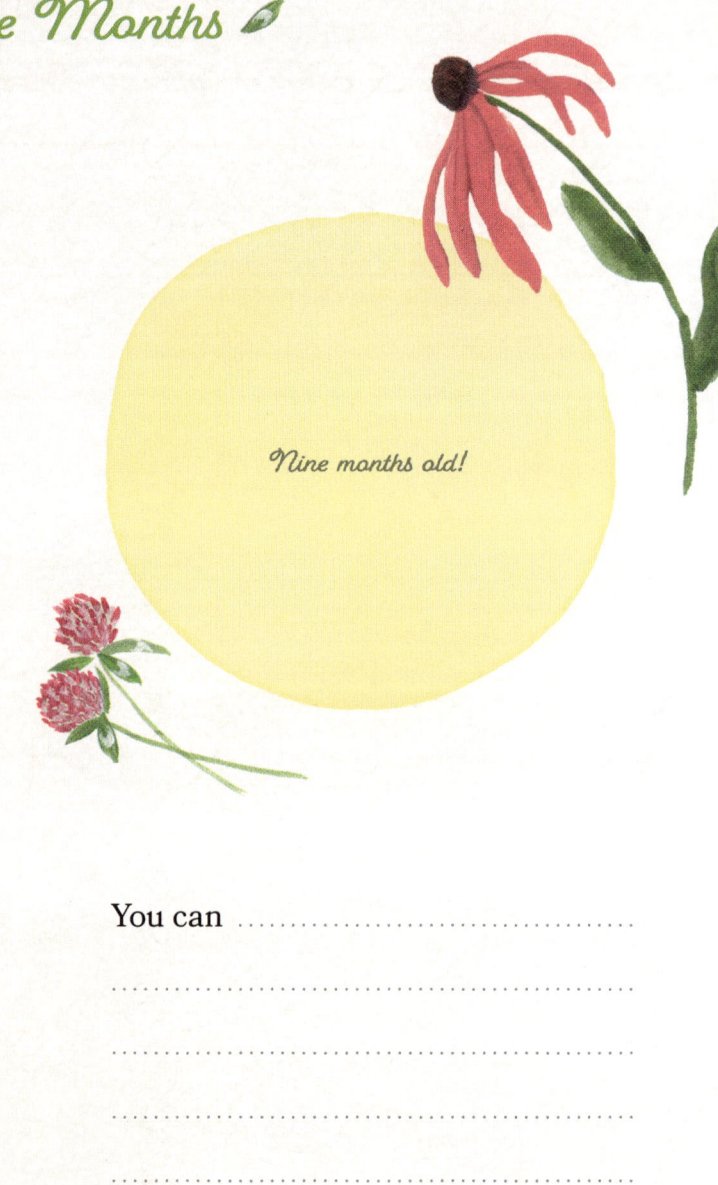

Nine months old!

You don't like ...................................
..................................................
..................................................
..................................................

You can ...................................
..................................................
..................................................
..................................................

Favorite book: .........................................

..................................................................

Favorite food: ..........................................

..................................................................

Favorite activity: .....................................

..................................................................

Favorite song: .........................................

..................................................................

Our family's favorite moments with
you this month: .....................................

..................................................................

..................................................................

..................................................................

..................................................................

..................................................................

*A favorite nine-month memory*

..................................................................

..................................................................

# Ten Months

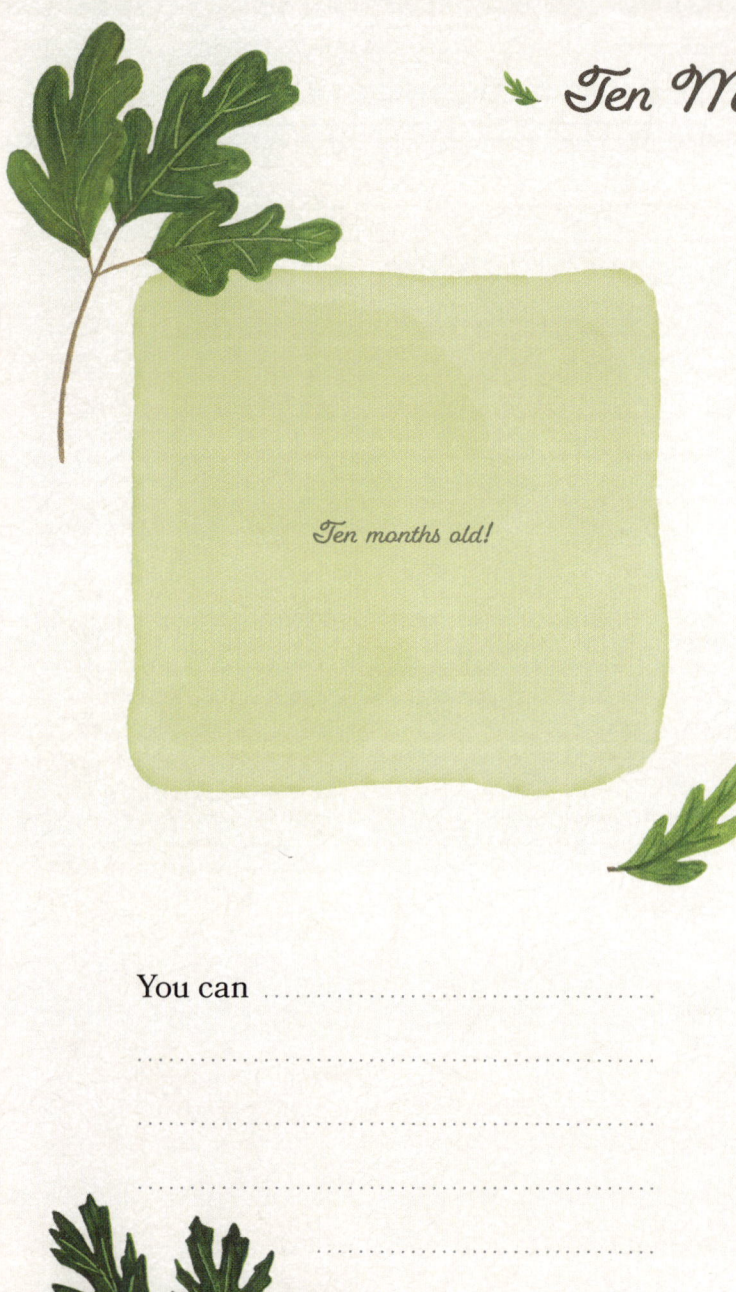

*Ten months old!*

On ........................................
you turned ten months old!

You weigh ....................................
and are ...................... inches tall.

You love ....................................
....................................
....................................
....................................

You can ....................................
....................................
....................................
....................................

You don't like ....................................
....................................
....................................
....................................

Favorite book: .................................  Favorite activity: .................................

Favorite food: .................................  Favorite song: .................................

*A favorite ten-month memory*

................................................................................

Our family's favorite moments with you this month: ................................

# Eleven Months

On ............................................
you turned eleven months old!

You weigh ..............................
and are .................. inches tall.

*Eleven months old!*

You love ...............................
............................................
............................................

You don't like .........................
............................................
............................................
............................................

You can ...............................
............................................
............................................
............................................

*A favorite eleven-month memory*

Favorite book: ..........................

Favorite activity: ..........................

Favorite food: ..........................

Favorite song: ..........................

Our family's favorite moments with you this month: ..........................

# Twelve Months

On .................................................
you turned twelve months old!

You weigh .......................................
and are ................. inches tall.

You love ........................................
................................................
................................................

You don't like ................................
................................................
................................................
................................................

You can .........................................
................................................
................................................
................................................
................................................
................................................

*Twelve months old!*

Favorite book: ......................................

Favorite food: ......................................

Favorite activity: ..................................

Favorite song: .....................................

Our family's favorite moments with you this month: ..........

*A favorite twelve-month memory*

# Happy First Birthday!

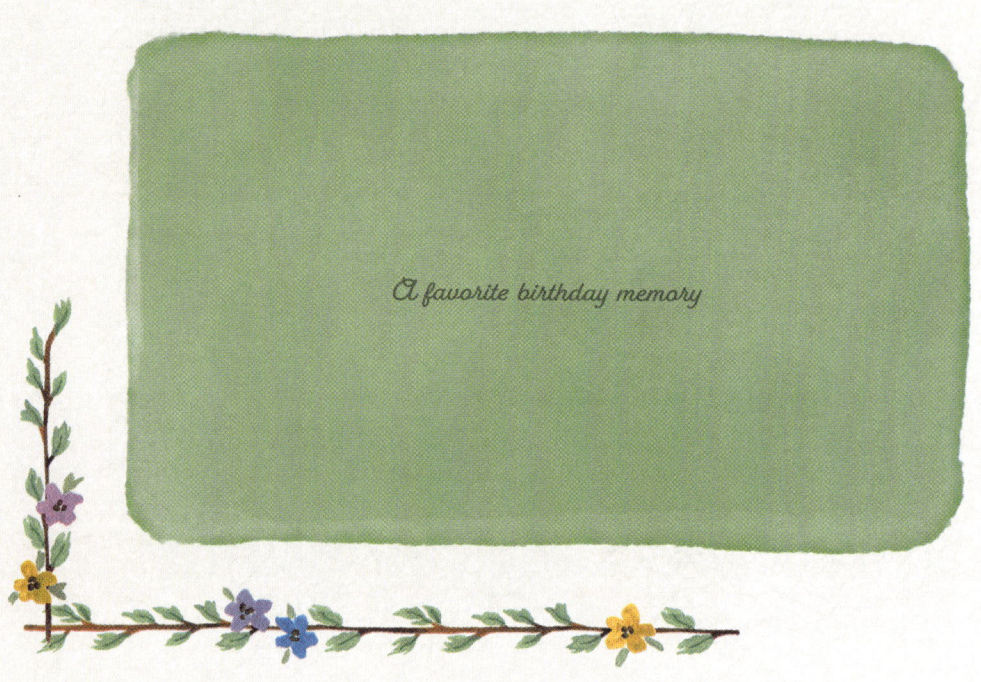

*A favorite birthday memory*

This is how we celebrated your very first birthday: ...........................................
................................................................................................
................................................................................................
................................................................................................
................................................................................................
................................................................................................
................................................................................................

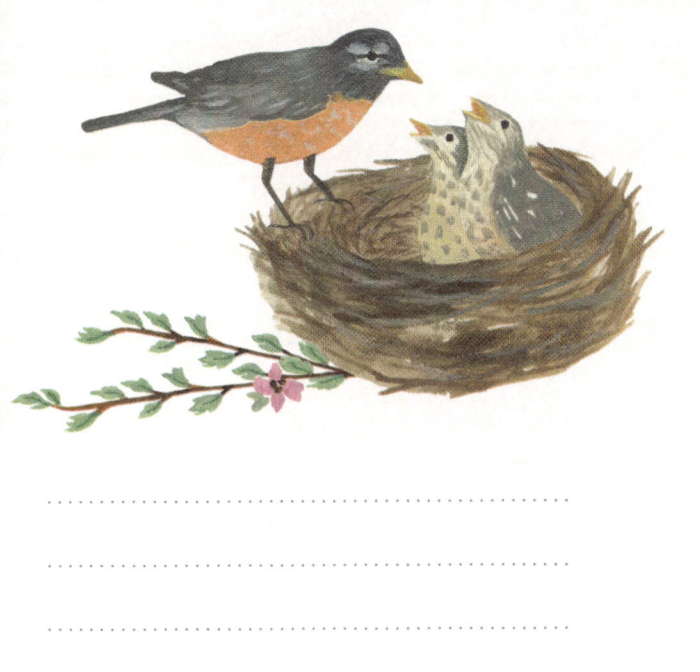
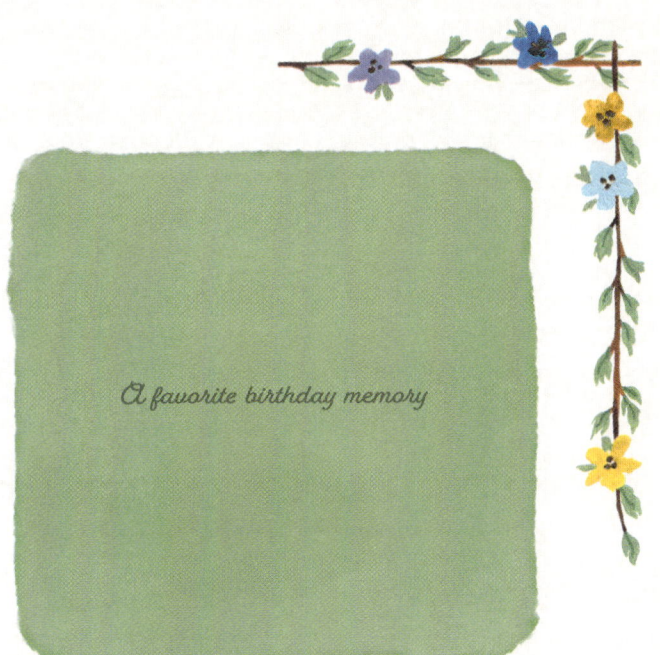

..................................................
..................................................
..................................................
..................................................

*A favorite birthday memory*

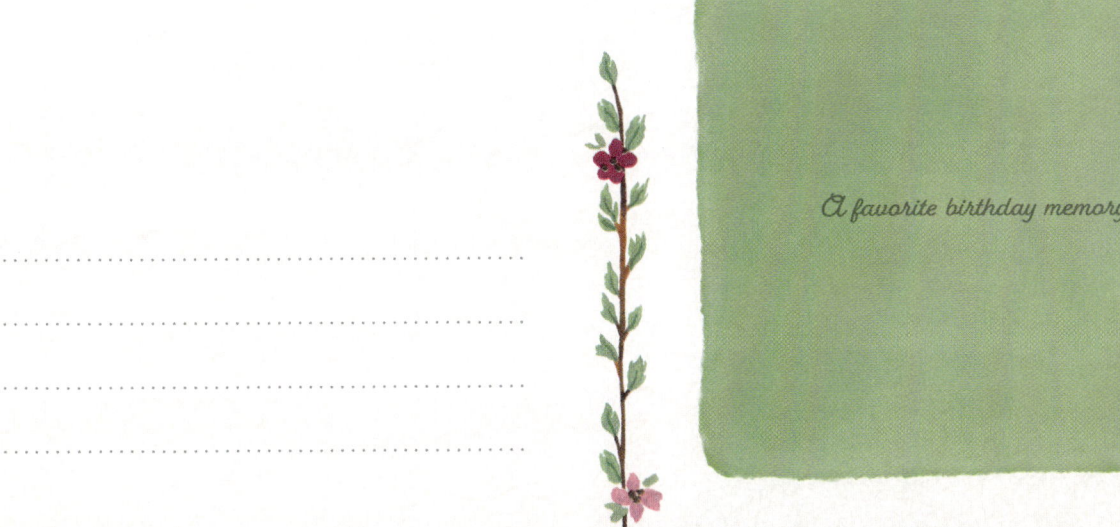

..................................................
..................................................
..................................................
..................................................

*A favorite birthday memory*

# A Year of You

Here are some things we've learned after your first year.

*A favorite photo from baby's first year*

You taught us .............................................................

You make others laugh by .............................

Times when you tried really hard: ............

Moments when you were kind: ............

Ways you wondered about the world: ........

Words you can say: ............................

# Wishes for You

Here are some wishes we have for you.

We hope you ............................................

We hope you learn ....................................

We hope you get ......................................

We hope you can .....................................

We hope you love ....................................

We hope you find .....................................

We hope you never forget ........................

We hope you become ..............................

We hope you grow ..................................

We hope you inherit ................................

45

# You're Two Cool!

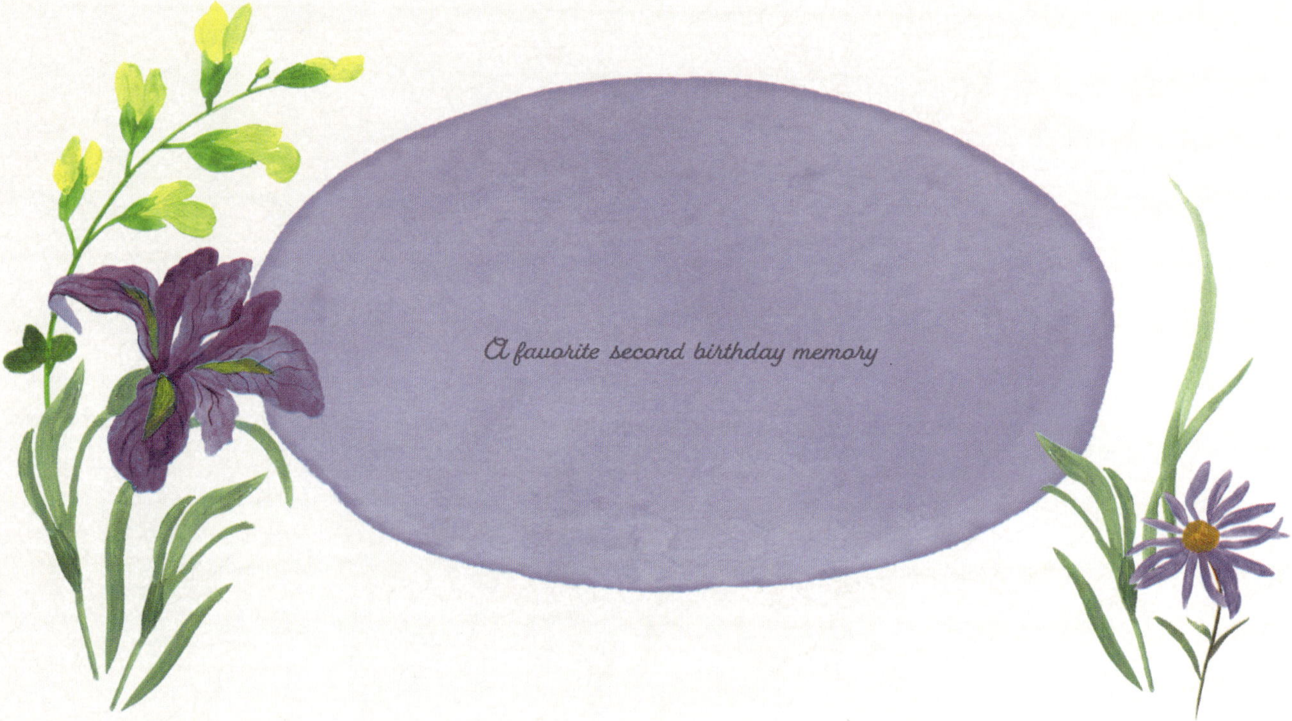

*A favorite second birthday memory*

This is how we celebrated your second birthday: ..............................................
................................................................................................
................................................................................................
................................................................................................
................................................................................................
................................................................................................
................................................................................................

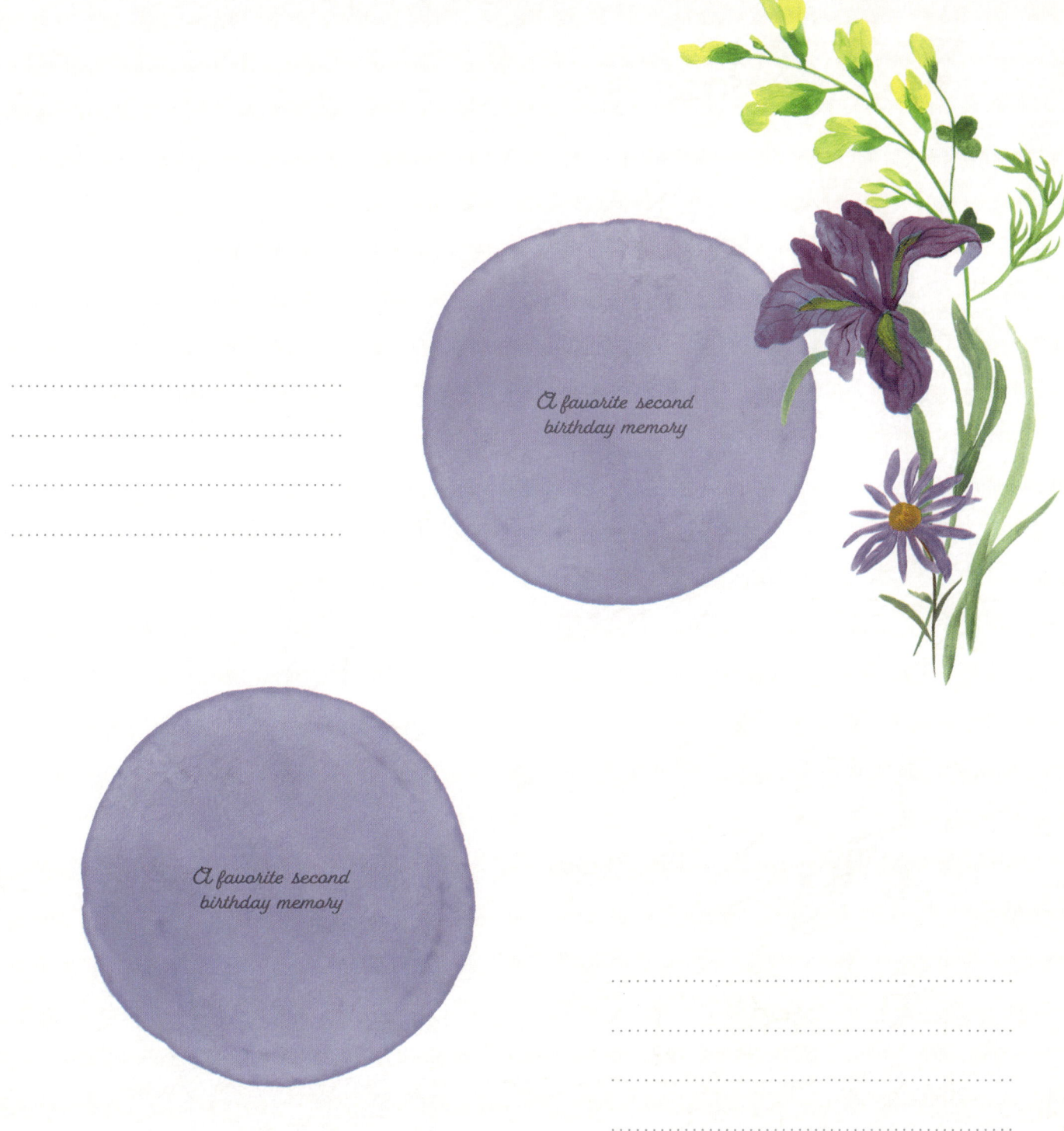

A favorite second birthday memory

A favorite second birthday memory

# Two Terrific Years

These are some highlights from your second year.

You taught us ..........................................

You make others laugh by ..........................

Times when you tried really hard: ..............

New friends you've made: ..........................

*A favorite photo from baby's second year*

Ways you explored the world: ....................

**Funniest things you've said:** ................................................
................................................................................
................................................................................

*A photo of baby laughing*

................................................................................
................................................................................
................................................................................

# Young, Wild, and Three!

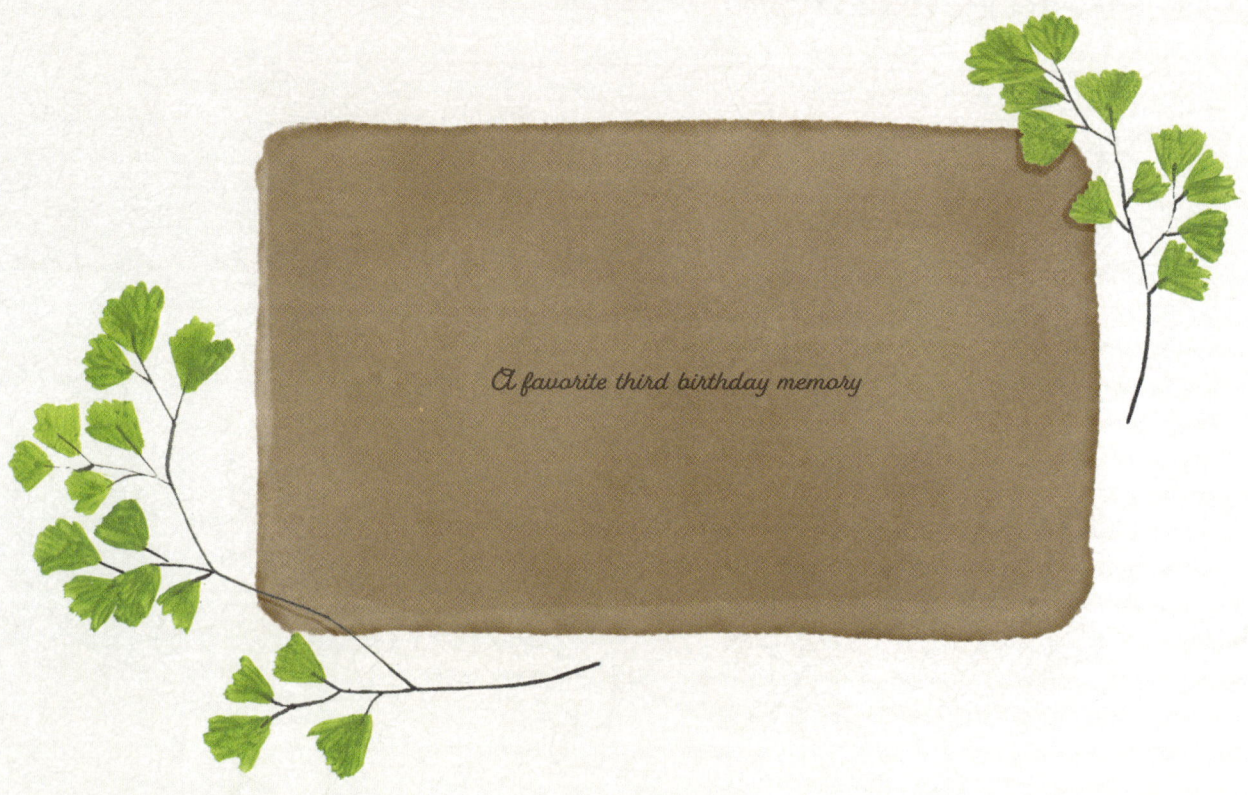

*A favorite third birthday memory*

This is how we celebrated your third birthday: ..............................
................................................................................
................................................................................
................................................................................
................................................................................
................................................................................
................................................................................

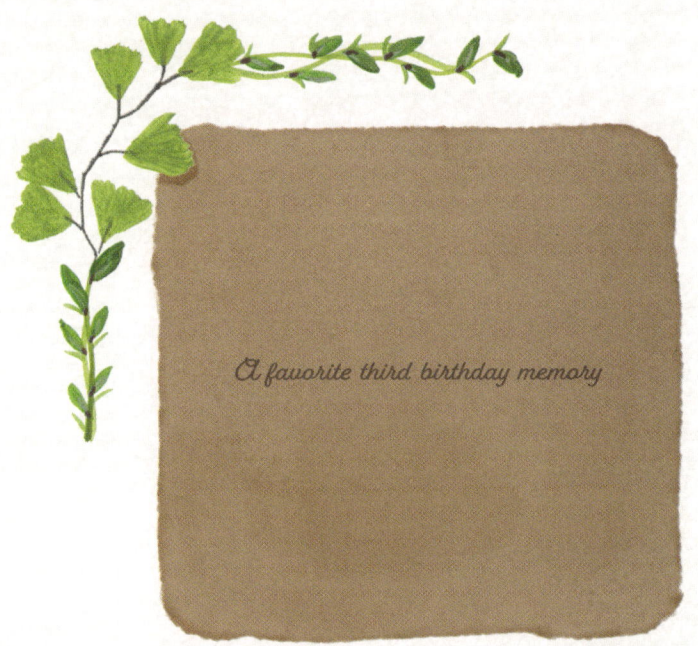

*A favorite third birthday memory*

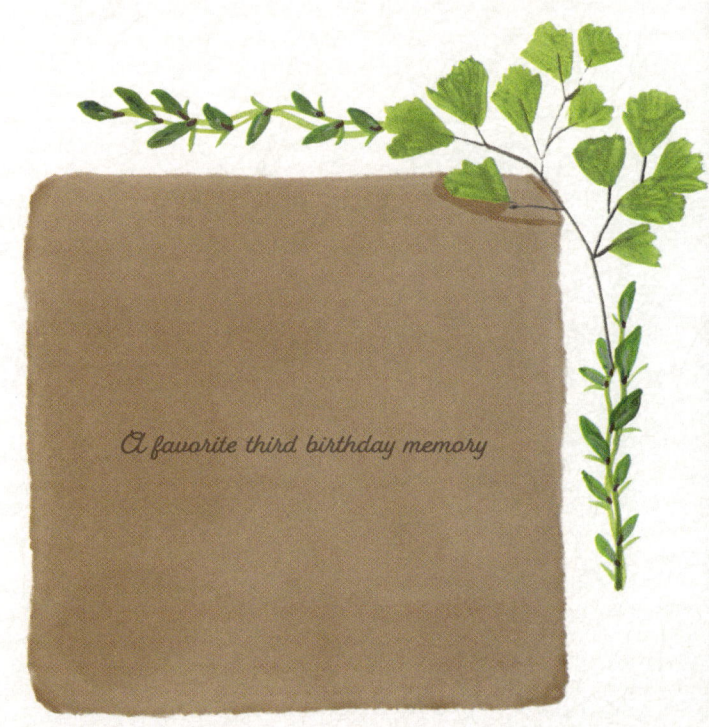

*A favorite third birthday memory*

# Three Years Strong

These are some highlights from your third year.

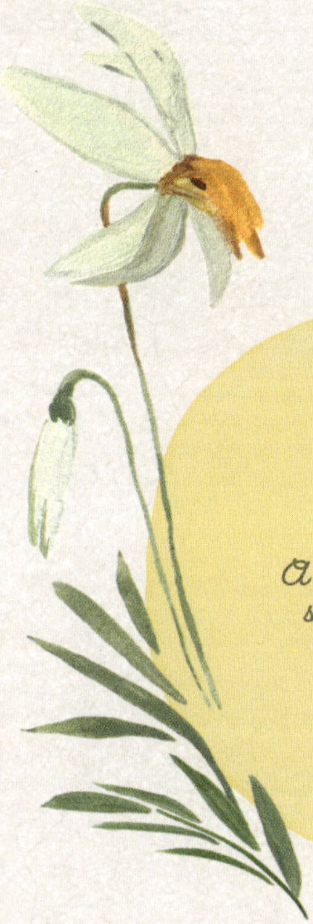

*A photo of baby doing something they love*

Now you are so good at ..................................
..................................
..................................

You are still learning ..................................
..................................
..................................

You love to go to ..................................
..................................
..................................

You taught us ..................................
..................................
..................................

You make others laugh by ..................................
..................................
..................................

Your favorite hobbies are ..................................
..................................
..................................

Some of your favorite people are ..................................................................
................................................................................................................
................................................................................................................

*A favorite photo from baby's third year*

................................................................................................................
................................................................................................................
................................................................................................................
................................................................................................................
................................................................................................................

# Favorite Places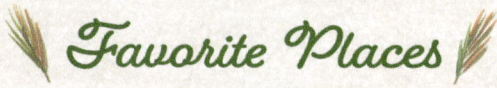

*A favorite place to snuggle*

*Baby's favorite place to play*

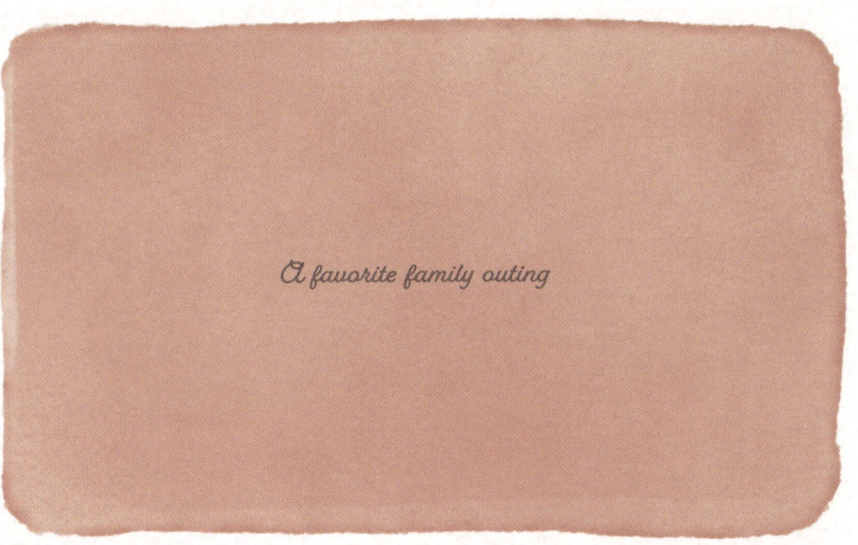
*A favorite family outing*

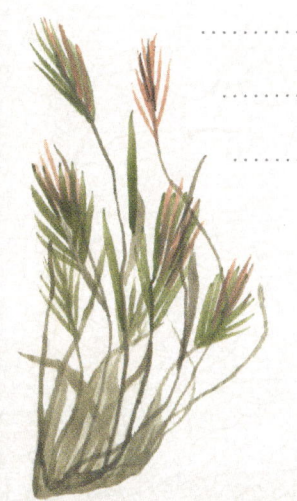
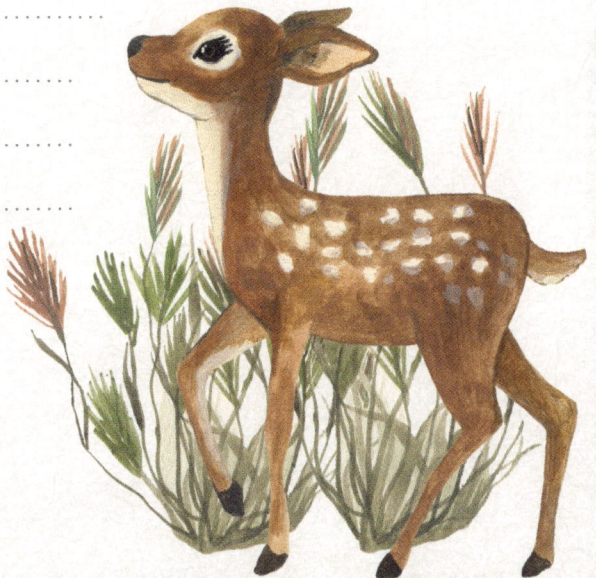

# Beginning with Books

Reading a book that
makes baby laugh

..........................................
..........................................
..........................................
..........................................
..........................................
..........................................

Snuggling with a story
baby loves to read at bedtime

..........................................
..........................................
..........................................
..........................................
..........................................

Reading a book Mom or Dad loved as a kid, too

Baby with all their books

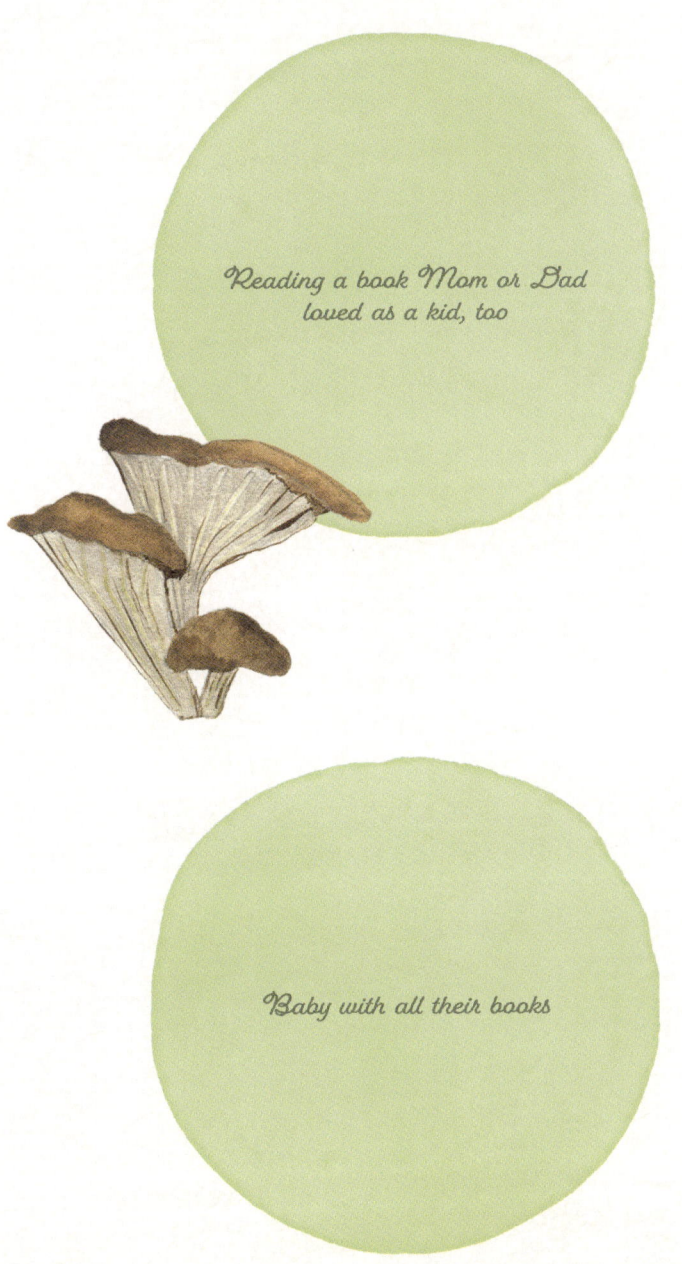
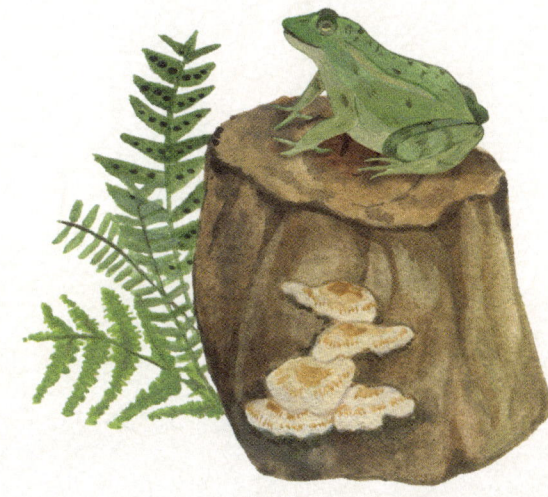

# Animal Friends

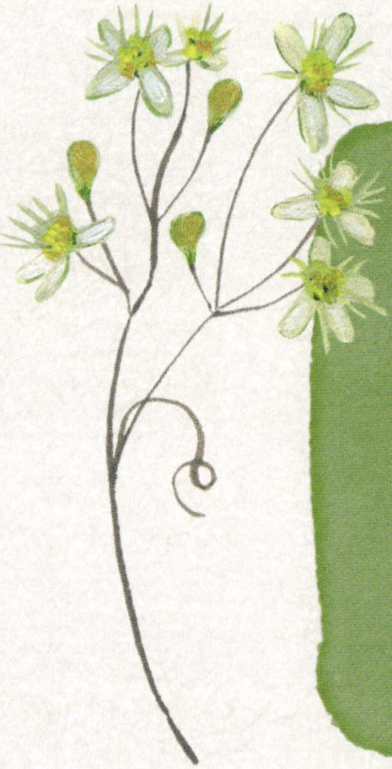

*Baby's favorite animal pal*

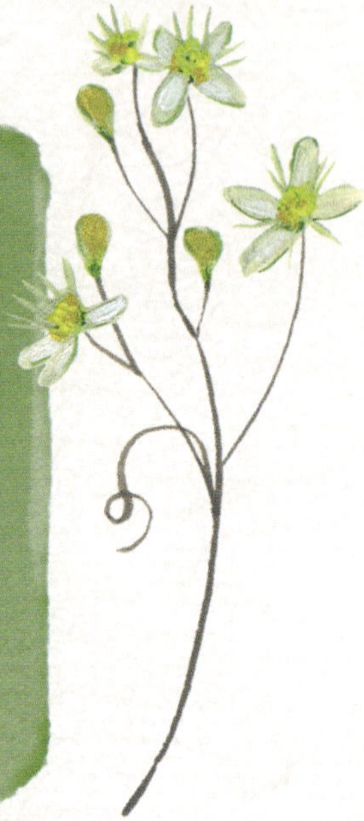

....................................................................
....................................................................
....................................................................
....................................................................

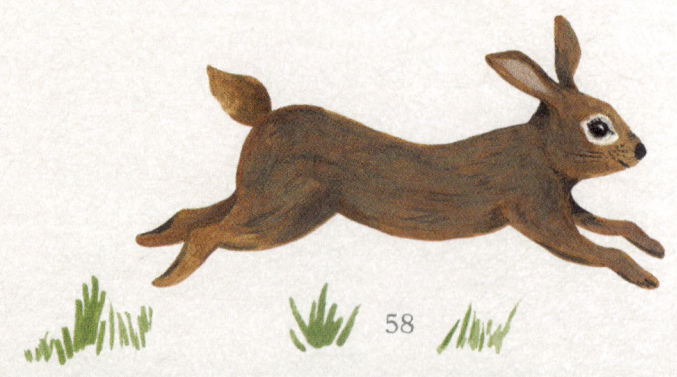

Baby with their stuffed animals

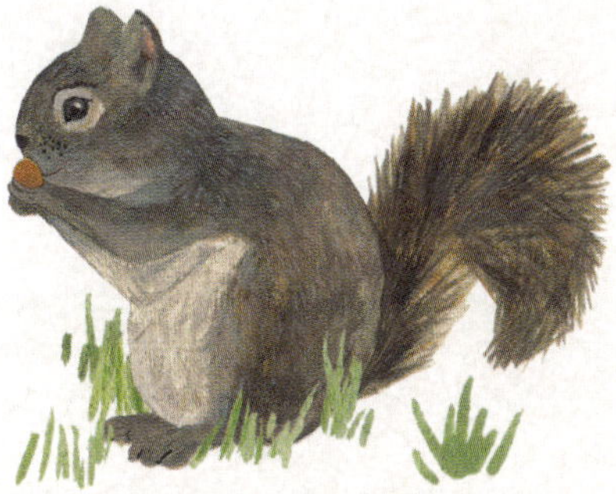

Visiting animals at the zoo

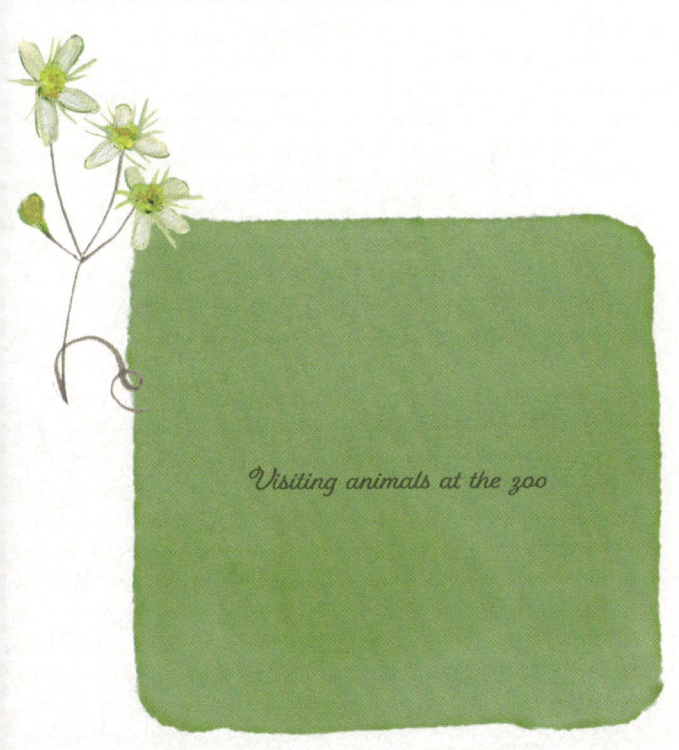

# Holiday Moments

*Baby's first holiday celebration*

*One of baby's favorite gifts*

*Our favorite way to celebrate together*

......................................................................................................
......................................................................................................
......................................................................................................
......................................................................................................
......................................................................................................

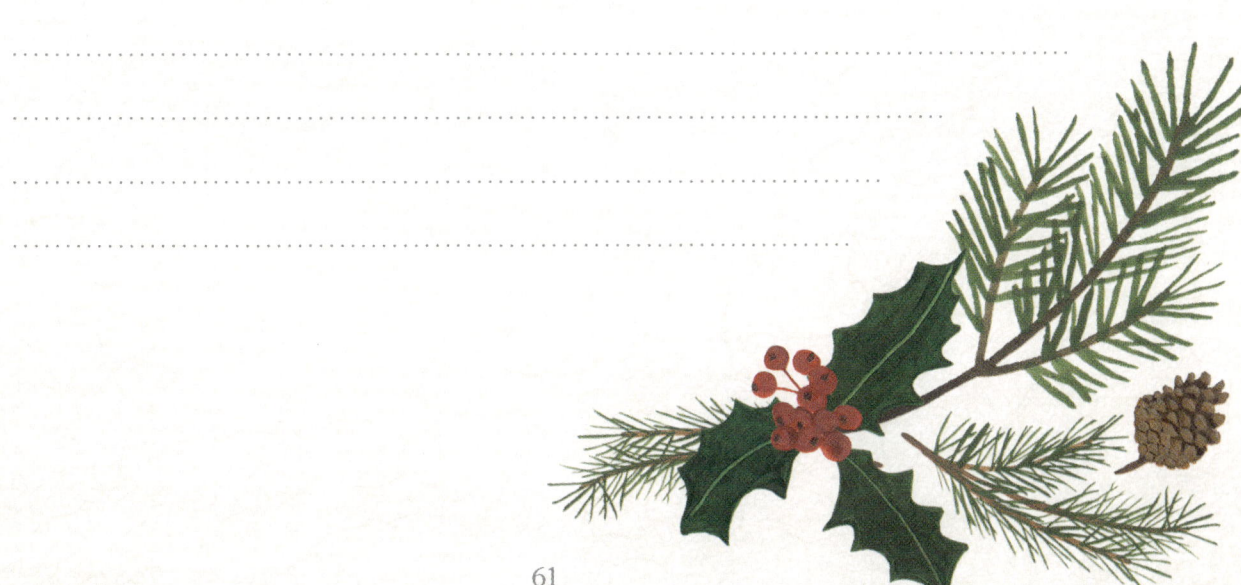

# A Letter to Future You

A letter to you as you continue growing and loving and exploring and learning...